ACCIDENT PREVENTION & FIRST AID

for use in playgroups

Compiled with the assistance of the British Red Cross Society

Cover photograph by Marian Pearson
Drawings by Sue Boud

ACCIDENT PREVENTION & FIRST AID

CONTENTS

	Page No.
Introduction	1
Parents are important	2
Emergencies	2
Frightened children	3
Fire drill	3
Health & Safety at Work Act 1974 and Health & Safety (First Aid) Regulations 1981	5
Check list for accident prevention and safety:	7
Premises	7
Group equipment & practice	8
Adults	10
Children	11
Toddlers and babies	11
Keeping the Accident and Incident Book	12
First Aid	13
First Aid boxes	14
First Aid A-Z	16
Emergency dental care	34
Coping with sick children	35
Childhood ailments	35
Childhood infectious diseases	35
Asthma	36
Meningitis	36
AIDS	37
Other problems	38
Emergency Information	39

INTRODUCTION

The best accident prevention is adequate supervision in a relaxed, happy atmosphere and the best first aid is calm, prompt action and comforting care.

Accident prevention is preferable to first aid but in spite of all precautions now and again someone will need to administer first aid of one sort or another in the parent and toddler group or playgroup. This booklet is intended as a simple ready reference. It contains advice to help you prevent accidents, information on what to do in an emergency and guidelines to enable you to decide when medical help is essential.

PPA recommends that a qualified first aider be present at every session. Everyone should know who this person is and in her/his absence a deputy should be appointed. Courses are run by organisations such as the St. John Ambulance Association and the British Red Cross. To find out about them, get in touch with your local branch, contact your nearest adult education centre, or ask your health visitor for information. Anyone involved in running a pre-school group and having a special interest in first aid would find such courses useful and interesting. In addition, any group employing staff is obliged to conform to the Health and Safety at Work Act like any other employer. (see p.5).

Your committee might like to plan a meeting for parents on basic first aid and you will find that organisations such as the Red Cross will often help by providing speakers. It is particularly important to have the correct instruction and practical demonstration for the emergency life-saving procedure of mouth-to-mouth resuscitation (the kiss of life).

One piece of advice repeated over and over again throughout this book is the importance of giving comfort and reassurance to the child who is hurt or in pain.

If there is a serious accident at your group, how will you cope? Will you feel too nervous to be of help? This is a problem that bothers most people and it is a normal reaction to feel shock yourself when a child is hurt. You may feel weak and wobbly at the knees, but take a deep breath, don't panic and make yourself appear cool, calm and confident. Immediate action will occupy your mind and help to maintain your self-control. You may surprise yourself by coping so well.

Parents are important

The comforting presence of a parent is as vital to the child as any medical treatment or surgery.

Parents are always very important people but in a situation where their child is injured or ill their presence is essential. If you arrive at a hospital or surgery with a child, the doctor may be unable to start treatment until the mother, father or guardian is present to give legal consent for any necessary treatment, such as stitches or blood transfusion. Other adults should not give their consent for such treatment. A frightened child needs his parents desperately and just can't understand why they are not there when s/he needs them so much.

It is very important to contact or fetch the mother or father when a child is ill or injured, but don't forget that they too will need comfort and reassurance to help them cope with the situation. If you take a child to hospital or surgery, be sure to stay until the parents arrive; in the hustle and bustle of a busy surgery, you may be the only familiar face. Once the parents arrive, you can act as a sympathetic friend because they are bound to be anxious or distraught. Children are not admitted to hospital if it can possibly be avoided, but parents may be upset and feel unable to cope with taking the child home, or may want the child home against medical advice. Your support will help them to act wisely and understand the situation.

Emergencies

If a sudden emergency should arise the child must be taken to hospital as soon as possible.

Send for an ambulance - dial 999.

Write down the following details for the hospital:

1. The child's name, age, address and telephone number.
2. The employer's name, address and telephone number (if the mother and/ or father are at work).
3. The name of the child's doctor.
4. Whether the child has had a tetanus immunisation and how recently, together with brief information on any known allergies.

Be sure that the person accompanying the child to hospital has these notes and can give an accurate account of the accident and the child's condition.

If you transport the child to hospital by private car, it is wise for someone left behind to telephone the hospital to warn them so that preparations for dealing with the case may be made. If transport is by ambulance, the driver will contact the hospital en route. If you can't get in touch with the parents, the police will contact them for you.

> **Always make sure that the records of your group are up to date so that you have the relevant details of each child readily available for such emergencies.**

Frightened children

If there is an accident in the toddler group or playgroup all the children will be shocked and frightened, particularly if there is an injury involving blood. Whilst the injured child is being treated, don't forget that the rest of the group will need reassurance too. Explain quietly and simply what has happened and what is being done about it, answer the inevitable questions and carry on with the session.

If there is a major disaster - a fire, a wall collapsing, a gas explosion - there will be an instant shock whilst everyone tries to grasp what has happened. In that instant, the adults must recover their senses first and get the children's attention immediately. Shout - say anything that comes to mind as long as it's an instruction: "Come here. Everyone follow me." Once you've given the instruction, repeat it and while you do, pull those lips into a smile; the children will be looking to you for a lead on how to behave and your example could save lives.

Don't let the children get more frightened than they are already or they just won't hear your instructions. If you have practised fire drill regularly, you can use it in an emergency; the children will know what to do and there will be something familiar and remembered in the midst of a dangerous and frightening situation.

Fire drill

Everyone in the group should have the opportunity to practise this twice each term. Since most groups have different children on different days, this may involve holding fire drill several times in succession.

Practise fire drill when the weather is not too bad. If there is a cloud burst, postpone the drill until later or wait for another day because there must be no pause for coats to be fetched. Don't let a chilly day deter you; the children will only be outdoors for a few minutes and can soon go back inside to get warm.

First of all you will need a fire alarm. It must be used exclusively for fire drill and it must make a loud arresting noise. The Fire Service recommends a 12cm (5") bell; it is a good idea to find out what your local infant school uses and copy them. Many of the buildings used by groups will already have a wall mounted fire bell and in this case you will need to use a special key to turn it on and off. Once outside the building, count the children and check with the register - which you must remember to take out with you. In toddler groups, make sure all parents are familiar with the procedure, as they remain responsible for their own children.

The Fire Officer will give advice on the best method of fire drill in your premises; invite her/him to your group and follow the instructions s/he gives. The Fire Officer will also show you how to use the fire extinguishers in the building and tell you if any particular doors should be kept unlocked during the session.

If you practise fire drill regularly, the children are less likely to be frightened if a real emergency occurs.

HEALTH & SAFETY AT WORK ACT 1974 AND HEALTH & SAFETY (FIRST AID) REGULATIONS 1981

All employers (including any playgroup committees which employ a leader etc) have a responsibility under the Health & Safety at Work Act to provide, so far as is practicable, for the health and safety of:

- employees
- children in their care
- rota parents and other helpers
- the public, in so far as they are affected by the group's activities.

All reasonable steps should therefore be taken to ensure that:

(a) the premises are kept safe to prevent risks to all users;

(b) the equipment is not dangerous and its manufacturer's instructions for use are followed;

(c) the adults working in the group are instructed in all matters of health and safety;

(d) all cuts, bumps and falls as well as other, more serious accidents are recorded in an Accident and Incident Book kept with the toddler group or playgroup records;

(e) fire precautions are observed.

Under the Health and Safety (First Aid) Regulations 1981 all workplaces must have first aid provisions.

As employers, toddler group and playgroup committees have a responsibility under these regulations for

(a) providing a first aid box for employees;

(b) seeing that each session has either a first aider or an 'appointed person' to take charge in the event of an accident,

(c) notifying all employees (eg through notices posted in conspicuous places) of (i) location of the first aid box and (ii) names of first aiders/appointed person(s),

(d) seeing that records of accidents to employees are kept.

The first aid regulations apply to employees only, but it is sensible and advisable to combine first aid arrangements for employees and non-employees. Contents of first aid boxes should follow Health & Safety Executive guidelines. A list of contents is provided on page 14.

> **It is a legal requirement if staff are employed that there is an APPOINTED PERSON at each session to take charge of any incidents and be responsible for the first aid box. Even if no staff are employed, this is still the recommended procedure.**

In order for a playgroup to fulfil its obligations under these two Acts, it is advisable that the committee appoints a committee member to take a special interest in safety and first aid. Her/his work could include:

(a) keeping an up-to-date list of group first-aiders and appointed persons;

(b) arranging first aid training for all interested adults but particularly the 'appointed person(s)';

(c) arranging for everyone working in the group to be made aware of safety policies and first aid provisions, not forgetting new playleaders and parents;

(d) regularly inspecting the Accident & Incident Book along with the committee;

(e) compiling a check list for accident prevention and safety and ensuring its regular use;

(f) notifying the committee of all matters requiring their attention.

There may, from time to time, be circulars from your local health authority or social services department or leaflets from health education officers relating to health matters which it would be a good idea to keep with this booklet for reference.

Local information, including information on training for Appointed Persons, can also be acquired from your PPA regional office or the Employment Medical Advisory Service. The Employment Medical Advisory Service is in the telephone directory under **Health & Safety Executive.**

SUGGESTED CHECK LIST FOR ACCIDENT PREVENTION AND SAFETY

No check list could cover every toddler group or playgroup situation, but this may act as an example to which you can make additions to suit your group.

Premises

Entrance

- Are doorways, stairs, locks, mats and steps safe or inaccessible?

Heating

- Are premises adequately heated and ventilated?
- Are radiators, pipes and fires guarded?
- Are heaters used in accordance with the manufacturer's instructions?

Fire

- Where are the fire extinguishers?
- When were they last checked?
- Do people know how to use them?
- Is there always free access to the fire doors?
- When was the fire drill last practised?
- Is the fire drill clearly displayed for parents, visitors and helpers?

Electric points

- Are these safe?
- Are plugs and leads inspected regularly?
- Where is the fusebox?

Other equipment in hall/play area

- What about chairs, tables and equipment (eg pianos) belonging to other organisations? Are they stacked or stored safely?
- Is dangerous litter left by other users (eg cigarette ends, ring pulls from drinks cans) removed before the session starts?

Kitchen

- Do electric cables trail from kettles or other electrical equipment?
- Where are detergents, cleaning fluids, matches and disinfectants kept?
- Do you have rules about children going into the kitchen and do all the adults using the group know about them?

Outdoor play space

- Are gates and fences childproof?
- Is there adequate adult supervision all the time the children are out to play?
- Is the play space inspected daily for broken glass, fouling by animals etc?

> **All faults in relation to premises (dangerous floors, faulty switches etc) should be reported to the owners and pointed out to all adults involved in running the group so that accidents can be prevented until such time as repairs are made.**

Group equipment and practice

Floor and floor coverings

- Are mats or rugs liable to slip or curl at the ends?
- Does the ground sheet and/or polythene sheet lie flat?
- Are spills mopped up quickly?
- Are toys picked up off the floor to prevent the risk of tripping over them?
- Is spilled sand regularly swept up to prevent slipping?
- Do you use a candlewick bedspread under the sandpit to limit the spread of spilled sand?

Tables, chairs, screens

- Do these stand secure?
- Are improvisations quite steady?
- What about adult chairs with open backs and trestle-type tables with faulty catches?

- Are large items like the folding bookcase and home corner anchored adequately?

Sand, water, dough, paint and plasticine

- Are dough and plasticine renewed often enough?
- Is the sand rinsed clean of dust and dirt regularly?
- Should water be changed more than once a morning and is cold water always put in before hot?
- Are the thickeners in paint free of fungicide?

Climbing equipment

- Are there broken spars, splinters, missing screws or bolts?
- Is there always an adult close at hand to supervise children using large equipment?
- Are ropes frayed or worn?

Toys

- Are they in good condition?
- Are the manufacturer's instructions observed?
- Are there too many little bits and pieces to be popped into mouths and ears?

Dressing-up clothes

- Could that evening dress trip someone up?
- How often are hats, wigs and clothes washed or cleaned?
- Are those heels high enough to cause a fall? Should they be permitted on the climbing equipment?

Glue, crayons, pencils, chalk
- Are they all non-toxic?
- Do you know of the danger of inhaling/swallowing pen tops?

Wheeled toys
- Are they safe and well-maintained?
- Is there a special area for these toys to avoid collision and interference with children engaged in other activities?

Woodwork
- Are tools of good quality and well looked after?
- Are tools available only with adult supervision?
- Are there enough vices or clamps to hold wood still?
- Is the bench sited well away from the main traffic areas?

Cookers
- Are the children allowed in the kitchen without supervision?
- If the cooker is used while the children are in the kitchen, is there continuous supervision?
- Are precautions taken after cooking whilst the cooker is still hot?

Storage
- How safe is the cupboard or storage area?
- Could articles topple off shelves?
- Are containers clearly labelled?
- Are substances which might be harmful to children (bleach, detergent) kept well out of their reach or locked away?
- Are flammable materials (meths, turps, gas cylinders) kept in secure storage out-of-doors?

Adults
Are handbags and shopping bags (with their often potentially dangerous contents) put out of the children's reach during the session?

- Should adults smoke? (In view of the recent evidence about passive smoking harming unborn babies, groups should discuss the subject carefully).
- Are cigarettes, lighters and matches kept out of sight and reach of the children?
- When lifting heavy objects are people encouraged to bend their knees, keep their backs straight and ask for assistance when necessary?
- Are you careful to prevent accidental scalding from hot drinks? (Mugs are safer than cups and saucers.)

Children
- Are shoe laces tied and buckles done up?
- Do anoraks have elastic at neck and waist rather than lethal laces?
- Is running madly around the room allowed?

Toddlers and babies
- Do you have a satisfactory place to park prams and pushchairs?
- Is there a safe place for the babies to play?

KEEPING THE ACCIDENT & INCIDENT BOOK

This book is used to record all cuts, bumps and falls as well as other accidents. It should be kept with the group's records and should be filled in promptly as soon as the injury has been dealt with. The important details to be recorded are:

- the full name of the casualty (adult or child)
- the date, time and place of the accident or incident
- the circumstances of the accident or incident
- a brief description of the injury sustained
- the name of the person who dealt with the incident
- the first aid treatment administered
- whether or not medical aid had to be sought and if so where and from whom.

It is essential to record all the information even in the case of minor injuries because on rare occasions some seemingly trivial accident may give rise to more serious symptoms later and your accurate notes may be vital.

Frequent accidents involving the same child or the same piece of equipment can also be a useful indication of the need for extra supervision of some activities or perhaps the re-positioning of equipment. Someone in the group needs to be responsible for checking the accident book regularly for indications of this kind.

If there is any likelihood of an insurance claim after a child (or adult) has been injured, the insurance company may require more details of the incident. Draw a rough sketch of the place of the accident (as in a road traffic accident) noting the positions of equipment and adult helpers.

Please remember that accidents do occur on group outings and it is just as vital to record all these in the accident book. It is a good idea to take the accident book with you, as well as the first aid kit.

> **It is essential to inform parents of any injury to their child no matter how slight.**

FIRST AID

First Aid falls into three categories:

1. Attending to minor cuts and grazes, always remembering that extra care and caution must be taken with other people's children. When in the slightest doubt, contact a parent and get medical advice.
2. The emergency measures we must take until trained medical personnel take over from us; we can prevent the injury or shock from getting worse by gentle and sympathetic handling.
3. The drastic life-saving action which must be taken at once by us, because waiting for medical aid might result in the death of a child:
   - if breathing has stopped
   - if the child is breathing, but unconscious
   - if there is severe bleeding
   - if there are burns
   - if poisons have been taken

All these are situations where a person trained in first aid must act immediately; mistakes could be fatal and medical help should be called without delay.

EMERGENCIES Dial 999

POSSIBLE EMERGENCIES
Remember to contact parent as soon as possible
GET QUALIFIED HELP

MINOR INJURIES
Remember to tell parents when child is collected

First Aid Boxes

List of Contents
Required under the Health & Safety (First Aid) Regulations 1981, amended 1990

Item	Quantity
Guidance Card	1
Individually wrapped sterile adhesive dressings (assorted sizes)	20
Sterile eye pads, with attachment	2
Individually wrapped triangular bandages	6
Safety pins	6
Medium sized individually wrapped sterile unmedicated wound dressings 10cm x 8cm (4"x3") approx.	6
Large sterile individually wrapped unmedicated wound dressings 13cm x 9cm (5"x3") approx.	2
Extra large sterile individually wrapped unmedicated wound dressings 28cm x 17.5cm (11"x7") approx.	3

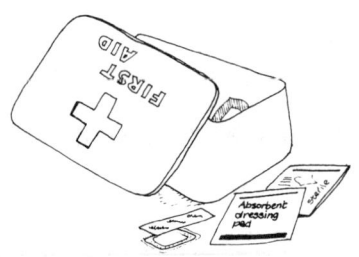

List of contents - travelling first aid kits
Required under the Health & Safety (First Aid) Regulations 1981, amended 1990

Item	Quantity
Guidance Card	1
Individually wrapped sterile adhesive dressings	6
Large sterile unmedicated dressing	1
Triangular bandages	2
Safety pins	2

Individually wrapped moist cleansing wipes

First aid boxes/containers should be waterproof and air tight as far as possible and identified with a white cross on a green background.
A playgroup first aid box may need additional articles, eg.
    A pair of sharp scissors
    A pair of tweezers
    A roll of non-allergenic adhesive tape (micropore)
    Packs of sterile gauze
    Crepe bandage
    Disposable waterproof gloves.

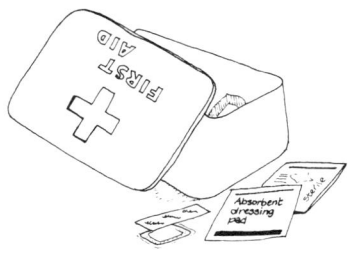

FIRST AID A-Z

Bleeding

Severe bleeding

Treatment:

- Where possible, wear disposable rubber gloves. This will reduce the possibility of any cross infection.
- In an emergency use direct pressure on the wound using your hand(s).
- If the wound is large, squeeze the sides of the wound together, gently but firmly, and maintain pressure.
- Lie the child down and, if possible, raise the injured part.
- Place a sterile unmedicated dressing over the wound and secure with a firm bandage (but not so tight as to cut off the circulation).

If bleeding continues, apply further dressing or pads and bandage firmly. Do not remove the original dressing. An improvised dressing can be made from any suitable clean material.

Treat for **SHOCK** (p31). Comfort and reassure.

REMOVE TO HOSPITAL IMMEDIATELY. CONTACT A PARENT.

Minor cuts and grazes

Use your discretion; some children need a cuddle first before treating the wounds. Wash the wound with warm water and soap. Dry. Apply an adhesive dressing or dry dressing, if necessary. Do not use antiseptic solutions or creams.

You may need to check the child's records to ensure s/he is not allergic to plasters, etc.

Bleeding from the tongue and lips

Sit the child down with head forward and inclined to the injured side. Control bleeding by placing clean dressing (crushed ice wrapped in this may help) over the wound and applying direct pressure with your thumb and fingers for about 10 minutes. Don't give the child hot drinks for 12 hours. If bleeding persists contact a parent and remove to hospital.

Nose bleed

Sit the child down with head well forward. Loosen tight clothing at neck and chest. Ask the child to breathe through the mouth while you pinch the soft part of the nose for 10 minutes. Have a small bowl or dark towel to catch any blood and ask the child to spit out any blood in the mouth.

Comfort and reassure; crying prolongs the bleeding. Keep the head well forward. If the bleeding continues, carry on with treatment for a further 10 minutes.

Gently clean with warm water. Do not let the child blow his nose, and avoid exertion. If bleeding persists, contact a parent and seek medical advice. Do not plug the nose.

Scalp wounds

These wounds bleed alarmingly, so be calm and comforting. Control bleeding by light pressure and cover with a dry dressing. Take the child promptly to hospital if stitches might be needed.

Internal bleeding

This may follow an injury such as a fracture, a crush injury or a sudden blow. There may be no outward signs. Internal bleeding is as serious as external bleeding.

Symptoms and signs may take some time to appear after injury. They may include pallor, shallow breathing, sometimes with sighing and yawning, restlessness and talkativeness, severe thirst. There may also be pain, tenderness or swelling in the area affected.

Treatment:

- Lie the child down.
- Check breathing passages are clear.
- Loosen constrictive clothing.
- Comfort and reassure.
- Treat for **shock** (p31).
- Stay with child.
- Check **breathing** (p19), **pulse** (p28) and level of **responsiveness** (p.30) every 10 minutes.
- Watch for vomiting.
- Do not give the child anything by mouth.

If the child becomes unconscious, place in the **recovery position** (p.28).

If breathing stops, follow the **ABC** drill under **breathing stopped.**

GET MEDICAL AID. CONTACT A PARENT.

Bites

Germs are harboured in the mouth of most domestic and wild animals (and humans). Dog bites are the most common bites and can produce deep puncture wounds. Any bite needs prompt attention to prevent infection.

Superficial bites

Wash wound with soapy water for 5 minutes. Dry. Cover with a sterile unmedicated dressing. Contact a parent and seek medical advice.

Serious wounds

Control bleeding by direct pressure. Apply sterile unmedicated dressing. Contact a parent and remove to hospital. Check whether the child has had the usual tetanus injections. Dog bites should be reported to the police.

Breathing stopped
Waste no time - seconds count. Get someone to call the ambulance.

Place the child flat on his back and follow this simple ABC drill.

A   For **Airway.** Ensure the Airway is open by tilting the head back, by placing one hand on the forehead and, with the other hand, using two fingers to lift the chin up and forward. This action will lift the tongue from the back of the throat.

B   For **Breathing.** Look, listen and feel. Put your face close to the nose and mouth of the child and also look along the chest line; you may see movement. If the above action does not re-start the breathing, you must breathe for the child. To do mouth-to-mouth resuscitation, maintain an open Airway and pinch the nostrils closed with finger and thumb of the hand that was holding the head back. Now place your mouth over the child's mouth, ensure a good seal and blow into the mouth. Watch the chest rise. (Do not over-inflate.) Remove your mouth and watch the chest deflate; take a fresh lungful of air yourself, and repeat the procedure. Check for a pulse.

C   For **Circulation.** Check the carotid pulse. This is situated in the hollow of the neck between the voice box and the adjoining muscle. If you find a pulse, then breathe for the child at a rate of 20 breaths per minute (1 breath every 3 seconds). If there is no pulse, then external chest compression will be needed. **This technique should be carried out only by those who have been fully trained in Cardiopulmonary Resuscitation (CPR).**

Once the child starts to breathe for himself, turn him into the **recovery position** (p.28).

ALWAYS TRANSFER TO HOSPITAL. CONTACT A PARENT.

Broken bones see fractures (p.26)

Bruises
A bruise is a discoloration of the skin because of bleeding into the tissue after a fall etc.

Aim to slow down the blood flow by cooling the injured area with a cold compress. If possible raise and support the injured part. Seek medical aid if there is any doubt regarding the extent of injury.

Burns and scalds

The treatment is the same for both burns and scalds.

Minor burns and scalds

Immediately place injured part under cold running water or immerse it in cold water for 10 minutes - longer if the pain persists. (Any cold harmless liquid can be used, eg milk). Gently remove any constricting items from the area, eg rings, watch, bracelet. Dress the area with a sterile unmedicated dressing.

If blisters form, do not break. Cover and get medical aid immediately.

Severe burns

Lie the child down. Remove constricting items, eg watch, bracelet, belt. Cool the affected area for 10 minutes or until the pain subsides. Deep burns are not quite as painful as superficial (reddening of the skin surface) or intermediate (reddening with blisters) as the nerve endings have been burned away. Dab dry. Cover the injured area with sterile unmedicated dressing. If this is not large enough, think of using an ironed pillowcase or sheet maybe. Treat for **shock** (p.31). If conscious give frequent measured sips of water. If unconscious place in **recovery position** (p.28).

REMOVE TO HOSPITAL. CONTACT A PARENT.

- **Do not** use adhesive dressings.
- **Do not** apply lotions, ointments etc.
- **Do not** break blisters.
- **Do not** remove clothing, unless covered with corrosive chemical such as bleach, or anything which is protruding from a deep burn as this will probably have been burnt sterile.

> **Advise parents that all burns in children, if larger than 1cm x 1cm, should be seen by a doctor.**

Choking

1) For small children

Back slapping:

Sit or kneel and lay the child along your thighs, head down over your knee. Support the child's chest with one hand and slap the child smartly between the shoulder blades up to 4 times, using the heel of your hand. With your other hand check the mouth carefully to see if the obstruction has been dislodged. If this does not dislodge the obstruction it may be necessary to perform the abdominal thrust. This attempts to force air out of a choking casualty's lungs. Because there is a possibility that the action required can damage underlying organs, abdominal thrust must be used only as a last resort after back-slapping has failed.

ABDOMINAL THRUST

Sit the child on your lap or stand the child in front of you, his back against your abdomen. Place one arm around the child's abdomen. Support the child with your other hand. Clench your fist and place it thumb inwards in the centre of the child's upper abdomen. Press your clenched fist into the abdomen with a quick upward and inward movement. Repeat up to 4 times.

2) For a baby

In babies much less pressure is used.

Back-slapping:

Lay the baby's head downwards with its chest lying along your forearm. Using one hand to support the head, with the other slap the infant smartly between the shoulder blades up to 4 times. Alternatively sit down and lay the baby face down along your thighs with the baby's head over the ends of your knees.

ABDOMINAL THRUST

Place baby on a firm surface on its back with chin up and head tilted back to open the airway. Place the first two fingers of one hand on the upper abdomen between navel and breast bone. Press with a quick inwards and upward movement. Repeat up to a **maximum of 4 times.**

If choking persists, call an ambulance or take the child to hospital. Follow **ABC** drill under **breathing stopped** (p.19).

Take extreme care when removing an obstruction from the mouth of a baby. There is always a danger of pushing the obstruction further down.

NEVER GIVE PEANUTS TO A CHILD UNDER SIX YEARS.

In all cases of choking contact a parent and seek medical advice.

Clothes on fire

As soon as it is possible, lay the child down. This helps to stop the flames reaching the face. Dowse with water whenever possible. Worry about any mess later; the child's life may be at risk. If getting water is going to take a long time, again lay the child down and smother the flames by using either a coat, rug or blanket.

- **Do not** use any man-made fibres as these melt and stick to the skin.
- **Do not** roll the child along the ground as this can cause burns to previously unharmed areas.

Treat as for severe **burns** (p.20).

Convulsions

In young children up to the age of 5, a raised temperature may cause a convulsion. These are called infantile or febrile convulsions. The raised temperature is usually an early sign of an infection, especially measles or an ear infection.

Aim to prevent the child injuring her/himself and cool the child. Ensure a good supply of fresh air. Loosen any constricting clothing. Clear a space and try to protect the child from further injury. Cool the child by removing most of its clothing; fan and sponge face with tepid water but do not allow to become chilled. The temperature must be brought down.

Contact a parent and seek medical advice.

At the end of the convulsion, place a child in **recovery position** (p.28).

Comfort and reassure child and parent.

If fitting continues for 10 minutes or more, or if the child is having recurrent seizures, telephone for an ambulance and notify the child's parents and GP.

Crush Injuries

The commonest crush injury is a squashed finger, which can be very painful. Wash off any dirt and apply a dressing if there is any bleeding. If there is blood under the nail or if you suspect a fracture, take the child to hospital.

Major crush injuries (eg leg caught under a falling object) are rare but if they occur, control serious **bleeding** (p.16) and dress the wound. Keep the child as still as possible. Treat for **shock** (p.31). Contact a parent and transport to hospital.

If the limb or part of the body has been trapped and crushed for as long as an hour, then no attempt should be made to release it. The build-up of toxic wastes in the blood is dangerous and could prove fatal by causing kidney failure. This child must be released by professionals.

Dislocations

Dislocated joints are very painful. Treat as **fracture** (p.26) by supporting the injured part in the position most comfortable for the child. Comfort and reassure. Contact a parent and transfer to hospital.

Electric shock

If possible switch off electricity at mains. If this is not possible, stand on some dry insulating material - wood, rubber, lots of newspaper - and use a non-conductive item such as a wooden broom to separate the child from the source of electric current.

Treatment:
- Check **breathing** (p.19) and **pulse** (p.28).
- If necessary, follow **ABC** drill under **Breathing Stopped** (p.19).
- If the child is breathing, but unconscious, place in **recovery position** (p.28).
- Treat any **burns** (p.20). (Remove the child first from the place of injury; water and electricity do not go together.)
- Treat for **shock** (p.31).

    REMOVE TO HOSPITAL IMMEDIATELY. CONTACT A PARENT.

Exposure to cold (Hypothermia)
There is a possibility that a baby left outside in its pram may become badly chilled; this should be avoided by bringing babies into the group during cold weather. Severe chilling can develop into **hypothermia**.

Signs and symptoms: the baby is quiet and drowsy; his cheeks look a healthy pink but his skin is deathly cold to the touch. The baby will often refuse food. Treat by warming up gradually. Remove wet clothing or nappy and replace with warm dry towelling or blankets. Remove to hospital. Do not use hot water bottles or massage the baby's skin.

Faint
A faint is a brief loss of consciousness caused by temporary reduction in the flow of blood to the brain. It is uncommon in young children. It may be the child's reaction to fright, pain, lack of food or exhaustion.

If a child faints or is very pale, giddy and weak, lay the child down with its feet raised. Loosen tight clothing at chest, neck and waist. Ensure supply of fresh air. Cover with a blanket. Keep under observation, checking **breathing, pulse** (p.28) and level of **responsiveness** (p.30).

Comfort and reassure on recovery. Inform a parent.

Foreign bodies in eyes, ears and nose
Large foreign bodies in eye
This is one of the times when you must restrict a child's movements. Do not let him rub his eye or the damage will be made worse. Sit the child on your knee

and firmly but gently hold his hands down. Never try to remove embedded objects or any foreign body in the coloured part of the eye. Place a light pad over the affected eye and take to a doctor or to hospital.

Small foreign bodies in the eye (eg sand, insects)
The tear ducts may do their job and wash out the foreign body after a few moments. If this doesn't happen, try irrigating the eye with tepid water. Do this carefully, tilting the head to the injury side and, using a jug, pour the water gently from the nose side, catching it in a bowl or basin. Two people are needed for this job, one to hold the child and place her hand firmly over the child's eye, the other to pour and catch the water. You may need to use the corner of a clean, damp handkerchief to gently wipe out the dirt.

If your attempts fail, cover the eye with a light pad, contact a parent and take the child to a doctor or a nurse.

TELL THE CHILD'S PARENT AT HOMETIME, NO MATTER HOW SLIGHT THE INJURY.

Foreign bodies in the ear
Do not probe. You may push the foreign body further in and make things worse.

Gnats and very small flying insects can create great noise when trapped inside the ear. Another First Aid measure is to try to float the insect out. Use tepid/luke warm water. Lay the child on his side with the affected ear uppermost. Very gently try to float the insect out by gently pouring in the water. If this fails, then contact the parent and remove to hospital.

Foreign bodies in the nose
Do not attempt to remove the object. Ask the child to breathe through the mouth. Contact a parent and remove to hospital. If an identical item is available, take it to the hospital as it may be useful for X-ray comparison.

Foreign body in wounds
Carefully remove any small foreign bodies from the surface of a wound, if they can be wiped off easily. Never attempt to remove an embedded foreign body. Apply direct pressure to the edges of the wound on either side of the foreign body. Place a sterile dressing around and/or over the foreign body and build up cotton wool in a crescent shape around the wound, extending the padding until

it is high enough to prevent pressure on the foreign body. Secure with a diagonally applied bandage. Make sure the bandage is not over the foreign body. Elevate the injured part if possible.

CONTACT A PARENT AND SEEK MEDICAL ADVICE.

Fractures

A fracture is a broken or cracked bone. Suspect a fracture if there is obvious deformity **or** severe pain and tenderness **or** inability or reluctance to move the affected part. Swelling and bruising usually follow later. After any fall (which does not render the child unconscious) let the child make the first move and do not dash and pick up the child; watch the child's movements first and enquire about pain, tenderness and swelling.

General treatment:

- Always treat difficulty in breathing, severe bleeding or unconsciousness first (see **Breathing stopped** (p.19), **Bleeding** (p.16) **Unconsciousness** (p.33)).
- Do not move the child unless absolutely necessary; treat all fractures in the position in which the casualty is found unless there is immediate danger to life.
- Steady and support the injured part with your hands.
- Use rolled-up blankets to maintain child in position.
- Arrange removal to hospital by ambulance.
- Contact a parent.
- Treat for **shock** (p.31).

If removal to hospital is likely to be delayed, immobilise the body with padding and bandages. The bandages must be firm enough to prevent movement but must not interfere with the circulation.

Fractures of the spine

A fractured spine is a serious injury because of the danger of damage to the spinal cord. The neck and lower back are the vulnerable sites. Movement may cause permanent nerve damage. If there is any suspicion of spinal fracture CALL AN AMBULANCE AND DO NOT MOVE THE CHILD UNLESS THERE IS ANY IMMEDIATE DANGER TO LIFE. DO NOT USE THE RECOVERY POSITION.

- Keep the head steady by hand.
- Place rolled-up clothing alongside the child for support.
- Cover with a blanket.
- Wait for the ambulance.
- Contact a parent.

Head injury

Most head injuries cause only mild concussion, but a few can go on to cause life-threatening compression of the brain.

Concussion or "brain-shaking" is a temporary disturbance of the brain with brief loss of consciousness, loss of memory from just before the injury and sometimes nausea and vomiting.

Compression is a serious condition usually caused by a skull fracture, in which the blood collects under the skull and presses on the brain. If not recognised and treated it can be fatal. It may follow soon after the injury or it may occur up to 48 hours later. The main signs to look for are increasing confusion, drowsiness or unconsciousness, continuing nausea and vomiting, weakness or paralysis of part of the body, unequal sized pupils.

> **Because brain compression is so dangerous, all head injuries should be taken very seriously.**

i) Loss of consciousness:

   Check **Airway, Breathing, Circulation** (p.19). Place child in recovery position. Call ambulance to take child to hospital. Call parents and arrange to meet them there.

ii) Drowsiness, confusion, persistent nausea and vomiting, unequal pupils or weakness of part of the body:

   Take child to hospital immediately. Call parents to notify.

iii) If child loses consciousness for only a few minutes or seconds and recovers completely to normal self, telephone the parents and inform them that the child will probably need to be admitted to hospital for observation overnight. (If parents unavailable to pick up child within an hour, take child to hospital or to GP for assessment.)

EVEN FOR THE MOST MINOR BUMPS IT IS IMPORTANT TO TELL A PARENT AT HOMETIME. WITHOUT CAUSING UNDUE ALARM, ASK THEM TO LOOK OUT FOR THE SIGNS OF COMPRESSION LISTED ABOVE AND TO TAKE THE CHILD TO A DOCTOR IF THEY ARE WORRIED.

Poisons

Check breathing. If stopped, follow **ABC** drill under **Breathing stopped** (p.19).

If the child is breathing, but unconscious, place in the **Recovery position.**

If lips or mouth show signs of burns from drinking caustic fluids (eg bleach) or acids (eg battery acid), give a **conscious** child water or milk to drink. NEVER ATTEMPT to make a child vomit; this should be done only under hospital supervision, if at all.

Remove to hospital immediately taking samples of any vomit and poison taken and empty containers, etc. Contact a parent.

Pulse

This reflects how rapidly and effectively the heart is beating. It is best felt as the **radial pulse** on the palm side of the wrist near the base of the thumb, or as the **carotid pulse** on either side of the neck just below the angle of the jaw. In children the normal pulse may be between 60 and 100 per minute, but more important is any change in the rate following injury.

In particular:

- following a head injury, a **falling** pulse rate may be a sign of brain compression,
- in cases of external or internal bleeding a rapid and **rising** pulse rate may be a sign of major blood loss.

Recovery position

You will find this mentioned often throughout the First Aid section and it is important to know how to place a child in the recovery position. Use this position when a child is unconscious, likely to become unconscious or in any situation when he must be kept lying still after an accident or injury.

DO NOT USE THE RECOVERY POSITION IF A SPINAL INJURY IS SUSPECTED.

Use of the recovery position ensures that the airway is kept clear, eliminates the very real danger of choking on vomit and prevents the tongue from slipping back and blocking the throat.

You might like to practise placing a child in the recovery position with a co-operative conscious child; it is much easier than it sounds.

To move a child lying on her/his back into the recovery position:

START AT THE HEAD, COME DOWN THE NEAR SIDE,
THEN UP THE FAR SIDE.

- Kneel alongside the child, level with the chest.
- Open the Airway - head tilt and chin lift and turn the head towards yourself.
- Take the arm nearest to you, keep it straight and place the hand palm up as far under the buttock as possible. (This is important; it makes the turn easier, and you will be less likely to cause any damage to the elbow joint.)
- Straighten the near leg (if necessary).
- Lift the far leg, by placing your hands under the heel and under the knee, and place it over the near leg, at the feet.
- Now place the far arm across the body so that the fingers reach the shoulders.
- Hold the hand/fingers in place by using the back of your hand whilst supporting the head and face.
- Position yourself about 6" (15 cm) from the child and place your other hand at the waist and take hold of a handful of clothing.
- Pull the child up onto your thighs and allow the child to rest there.
- Readjust the head and airway.
- Place the uppermost arm out to support the upper trunk.
- Pull the top leg up by placing your hand in the crook of the leg.

- Gently move back and let the child settle. The stomach should not be in contact with the ground.
- Check that the far arm is out from under the child. If it is not, gently ease it out by pulling at the shoulder. Once in position, this will stop the child from rolling back.
- Go back to the head. Check and open the airway if necessary.
- Finally shake gently at shoulders and hip to ensure they are stable.

Stay with the child. Treat other injuries. Treat for **Shock** (p.31).

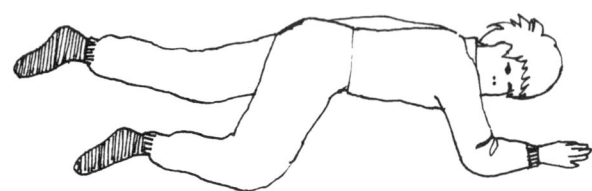

Responsiveness

To assess levels of responsiveness check eyes, movement and speech. This is a very good method of monitoring changes in the level of consciousness.

Eyes	Are they open?
	Do they open on command?
	Do they open to painful stimuli?
	Do they remain closed?
Movement	Does the child move on command?
	Does the child respond to painful stimuli?
	Is there no response at all?
Speech	Is conversation normal?
	Is the child confused?
	Are the words inappropriate to the question?
	Does the child make incomprehensible sounds?
	Is there no response at all?

The above monitoring checks should be done at least every ten minutes, and a log should be kept. These records, in serious cases, can be handed to the ambulance people when they arrive, who will in turn pass them to the doctor.

Shock

This is a condition of general weakness resulting from some injury which has reduced the volume of blood or fluid in the body. It is a serious condition as the loss of circulating blood may mean that there is insufficient oxygen reaching the brain. The main causes are severe **Bleeding** (p.16) and **Burns** (p.20). Heart attacks and severe diarrhoea and vomiting can also cause shock. All injuries can produce shock in a milder form.

The body reacts to shock by diverting more blood to the vital organs - brain, heart, kidneys - and less to the skin.

Treat for shock in all injuries:

- Look for and treat cause - **Bleeding** (p.16), **Fracture** (p.26), **Burns** (p.20), etc.
- Reassure and comfort.
- Place in resting position - lying down with feet raised; do not move unnecessarily.
- Keep warm with a blanket; DO NOT USE HOT WATER BOTTLES.
- Loosen tight clothing.
- Observe **Breathing, Pulse** (p.28) and level of **Responsiveness** (p.30).
- DO NOT GIVE FOOD OR DRINKS BY MOUTH. (Moisten lips only if patient is thirsty).

Contact a parent. Remove to hospital if injury warrants this.

Splinters

Wood splinters embedded in the skin are common in young children at play. *Remove with tweezers.*

First clean the area around the splinter with soap and water. Sterilise the tweezers by passing through a flame. Allow tweezers to cool. Gently try to pull the splinter out by holding the tweezers as near to the skin as possible, gripping the splinter and pulling it out in the opposite direction from its entry. If unsuccessful, contact a parent and seek medical advice.

Always check that the child is fully protected against tetanus.

Sprains and strains

A *sprain* is an injury which occurs at a joint when the surrounding ligaments and tissues are wrenched. A *strain* is an overstretching and sometimes tearing of a muscle. They may be difficult to distinguish from a **Fracture** (p.26).

Signs and symptoms include pain increased by movement, tenderness, swelling and later bruising.

Treatment should follow the RICE method:

- *Rest* - keep the affected part steady and supported in the most comfortable position.

- *Ice,* if available, can be applied immediately.

- *Compress* - compress the injured part. This is accomplished by applying cotton wool around the injury, and securing in place with a bandage. The bandage should be firm but not so tight as to cut off any circulation. This treatment will help to counteract any swelling.

- *Elevation* - raise the affected area if possible.

Contact a parent and seek medical advice.

If in doubt, treat as a **Fracture** (p.26).

Stings

These can be very frightening to children. Remember to comfort and reassure. If a bee sting is still embedded in the skin, attempt to remove, without breaking poison sac, using a pair of tweezers. Hold tweezers as near to the skin as possible. Apply a cold compress to relieve pain and swelling. If pain and swelling persist or increase, advise parents to seek medical advice.

Some children and adults are allergic to certain stings and have serious reactions. In the case of a generalised rash after a bee-sting, take the child to hospital immediately and contact the parents.

Stings inside the mouth may cause swelling resulting in breathing difficulties. In both these cases, arrange immediate removal to hospital. If possible give a child who has been stung inside the mouth an ice lolly or some ice cubes to suck or a drink of cold water.

Swallowed objects

Most small smooth objects are unlikely to damage the intestines or cause choking and if not too big they will pass right through the digestive system. If in doubt, seek medical advice.

Sharp objects such as pins, needles, nails and even pen tops can damage the intestines. In this situation do not give any food or drink. Contact a parent and transport the child to hospital. Take a similar object if possible to show the doctor.

Unconsciousness

Unconsciousness is the result of an interference with the functions of the brain. There are many causes - head injury, convulsions, poisoning, severe shock, etc.

Treatment:

- Check breathing - if necessary follow **ABC** drill under **Breathing stopped** (p.19).
- Ensure open airway.
- Treat serious wounds and severe **Bleeding** (p.16).
- Loosen tight clothing at neck and waist.
- If breathing normally and no suspicion of spinal injury, place in **Recovery position** (p.28).
- Monitor breathing, **Pulse** (p.28) and level of **Responsiveness** (p.30).
- Cover with a blanket and place one underneath if possible.

CONTACT A PARENT. REMOVE TO HOSPITAL.

NEVER leave an unconscious person alone. DO NOT attempt to give food or drink.

Winding

This is caused by a blow or fall on to the stomach. The child is momentarily unable to get his breath. It's a frightening experience so comfort the child and let him sit quietly on your lap for a while. It may help gently to massage the upper abdomen area. Loosen any tight clothing at neck, chest and waist.

EMERGENCY DENTAL CARE

(Advice supplied by the District Dental Officer, Coventry Health Authority)

Baby teeth If knocked out, leave out.

Advise parents to take the child to a dentist to check that no fragments of tooth are left in the gums.

Adult teeth If knocked out, these can be successfully replaced if the root is intact.

ACT QUICKLY

Always hold the tooth by the crown, *NEVER* the root.

Rinse off any dirt under a running tap; *NEVER* brush the root or use anything other than water.

Holding the crown, place the tooth back in the socket and take the child to the dentist.

If uncertain, place the tooth in milk or get the child to hold the tooth in his/her cheek and take the child to a dentist.

NEVER allow the root to dry.

NEVER wrap the tooth in tissue.

If the tooth is still in place but the crown is broken, advise parents to take the child to a dentist, who can usually build the crown up to its normal shape, size, and colour if the root is undamaged.

Do not delay in seeking care.

All general dental practitioners have arrangements to provide advice and, if necessary, emergency care for their regular patients outside their normal working hours.

COPING WITH SICK CHILDREN

Childhood ailments and the ill child

Playgroups are not suitable, enjoyable places when a child is ill. An ill child may be unable to tell you what is wrong or identify the position of any pain, and may be most uncooperative. Be extra patient and gentle.

A child who is unwell at the group should be taken home, so contact a parent. Give the parent full details of the child's symptoms so that the parent can decide if the child needs to be seen by a doctor. If the parent is unavailable, try to get the child to lie down in a quiet corner with an adult sitting close by.

Young children are susceptible to many illnesses and infections; where children are in close contact with one another infections can easily spread. There is no way to prevent this and children gradually build up an immunity to the common infections such as common cold, tonsillitis, ear infection.

Childhood infectious diseases

The common childhood infectious diseases are chickenpox, whooping cough, mumps, measles and rubella (German measles). Children should not attend playgroup when they have any of these infections. A useful list of incubation periods and time needed away from the group is provided in the PPA register and in PPA Guidlines or may be obtained from your health visitor or clinic.

Try to keep a note of the immunisations and infectious diseases each child has had and encourage parents to do so too. Also encourage parents to find out about immunisations against the serious infections - measles and whooping cough - if their child has not already been vaccinated.

Inform parents when one particular infectious disease seems to be "going round" your group, especially rubella which can be a danger to mothers in early pregnancy.

Keeping a stock of health education leaflets at the group will mean you always have information for parents at hand. These can easily be obtained from your local health education centre, health visitor or clinic.

Asthma
Mild to moderate asthma:

- child complains of feeling short of breath (breathing rapidly or panting).
- child is wheezing.
- child is short of breath at rest.

These three are usually combined with a cough.

Telephone parents and ask them to remove child for assessment as soon as possible.

If unable to contact either parent or emergency contact number within one hour, or if the child deteriorates at any time, contact the GP.

Moderate to severe asthma:

- child is distressed with shortness of breath.
- child short of breath while speaking (gasping for breath between words).
- child unable to get out of chair.
- child has blue lips, blue around the mouth.
- child is drowsy or abnormally quiet.
- child becoming exhausted.

Check to see if child has medication. (Some children have an aerosol inhaler or nebulizer.)

Get the child to fresh air.

Sit the child down and make him/her comfortable. The child may feel easier if sitting forward slightly.

If symptoms persist, contact parent. If parent not available within 5 minutes, contact GP or take the child to the GP or hospital.

Meningitis
If a child with fever shows the following symptoms:

- is abnormally drowsy or confused
- complains of headache

- complains that light hurts his or her eyes
- has a generalised rash (not obviously measles etc)
- has neck stiffness,

unless parents are immediately available, take child to hospital or ask to see the child's GP urgently. Meningitis is not common but it is an emergency in children as the disease progresses very rapidly.

The AIDS virus

The AIDS virus is carried in infected bodily fluids and is usually transmitted by sexual intercourse with an infected person or by using infected syringes and/or needles for injections. The virus is not spread by normal social contact, coughing, sneezing, sharing washing and drinking facilities or using the same lavatory.

A child with AIDS does not pose a threat to other children but may be at risk from them, as such a child has no defence against ordinary childhood infections and may often be too ill to attend the group. You will not necessarily know if a child or an adult in your group is HIV positive or has AIDS. Normal hygiene precautions will, however, prevent the spread of AIDS and of other blood-borne diseases.

It is important to ensure:

- That cuts or open wounds are covered with sticking plaster or other dressing, particularly if there is a risk of contact with other people's blood or other bodily fluids.
- That any spillages of blood, vomit or excrement are wiped up thoroughly. Materials should then be flushed away down the lavatory and floors and other affected surfaces disinfected using bleach diluted according to the manufacturer's instructions.
- That tooth brushes are not shared.
- That the first aid box includes disposable gloves.
- You wear disposable rubber gloves whenever possible when dealing with cuts, vomit and excrement.

Other problems

There are several other conditions that can easily be spread by close contact among children. They include the viruses and bacteria which usually cause diarrhoea and vomiting, conjunctivitis and impetigo and parasites like scabies, head lice and worms. Once the child has started treatment and is well, there is no reason for him to be excluded from the group but, of course, a pre-school group is no place for a child with diarrhoea and vomiting. If a child in your group has head lice, it is a good idea to ask the health visitor to come and check all the children in the group, but you will need to get parental permission for this inspection.

Although a sick child should not be present in the group, some illnesses develop very quickly and a child who arrived looking and feeling perfectly well may need help before the end of the session.

EMERGENCY INFORMATION

Date filled in _____

Nearest telephone _____

(Keep coins/cards for telephone box or keys of office in or near first aid box. Make sure everyone knows where they are. Is the phone accessible outside normal hours, eg for parties/open evenings/fundraising events?)

Ambulance   )
Police   )   **DIAL 999**
Fire Brigade   )

Nearest transport (eg taxi) _____

_____

Nearest Accident and Emergency Department _____

_____

Nearest Doctor's Surgery _____

_____

Police Station _____

_____

_____

Social Services Department _____

_____

Health Visitor or Clinic _____

_____

Fire Prevention Officer _____

_____

Area Health and Safety at Work Executive Officer _____

_____

Local St. John Ambulance/Red Cross _____

_____

Other important telephone numbers _____

_____

_____

_____

_____

**THIS INFORMATION COULD BE VITAL.
SET UP A SYSTEM FOR CHECKING AND UPDATING IT ON A
REGULAR BASIS.**

THIS PAGE HAS BEEN LEFT BLANK FOR YOUR OWN NOTES